Sugar Detox Plan

Crush Your Sugar Rush

With This 10-Step Sugar Free Diet

Authored By

Stephany J. Greene

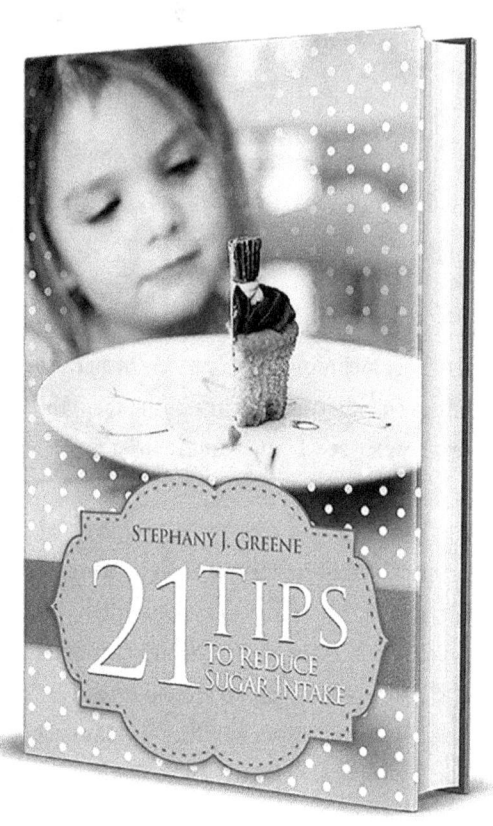

<u>YOUR FREE BONUS BOOK:</u>

"21 Tips to Reduce Sugar Intake"

Get it at:

<u>http://stephanygreene.site/free-ebook/</u>

About the Author

Stephany J. Greene is a young dietician and author from the state of California, who devoted her life to helping others become healthier. What other way to do that, than to write stories to actually achieve that? She has written multiple dieting books. Her published books have been well-received by a wide audience and even rewarded with a best-seller achievement! Learn more about Stephany by visiting her author website:

http://stephanygreene.site

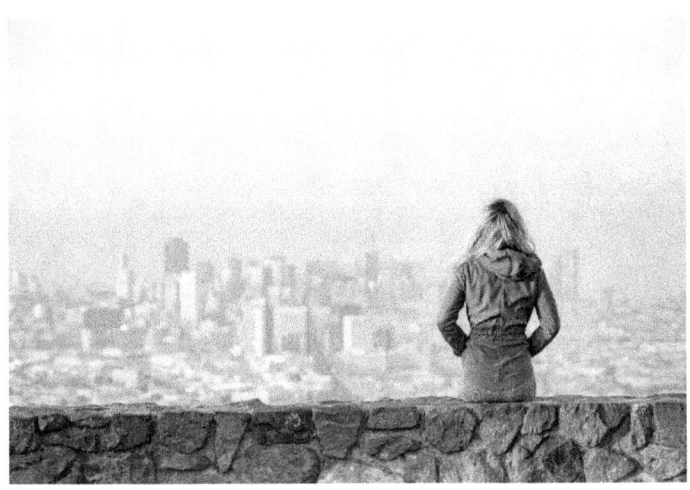

Table of Contents

Introduction

You've likely heard about the popular sugar detox diet. It's a three-week to month long eating program said to free you of a yearning for sweets (where sugar is commonly found) and assist you in adjusting your glucose levels. Its objectives are simple: to get you out of the desiring cycle and to help you maintain a healthy weight.

It is also an application of "instinctive eating," a diet technique that involves doing away with a specific food for a predefined timeframe before reintroducing it to see how your body responds.

In the case of sugar detox, you deprive the body of sugar for three weeks to a month, then you reintroduce sugary foods to see if you still crave them as strongly as you did before the diet.

Sugar detox plans persuade you to abstain from anything that transforms into glucose within your body. This includes biscuits and doughnuts, as well as most organic produce, low-fat dairy, and refined grains. By removing these common foods, the diet enables an individual to get out of a cycle of desire and adjust their body's glucose levels, which has a positive effect on vitality, weight, and rest, among other countless advantages.

You might think that you can't get through the day without Red Bull or sugar-laced doughnuts for a quick "buzz" of energy, but would you really say that this keeps your body maintained in the long term?

That early afternoon Red Bull, candy, or sugar-stacked goodie sets you up for a continuous cycle of awful eating and sluggishness.

This book is all about getting rid of sugary foods and drinks, and adopting healthy lifestyle. We will go over an entire detox plan and will introduce you to new ways of eating!

Don't forget to claim your own copy of the free bonus book I wrote (over at http://stephanygreene.site/free-ebook/), where you can find 21 more useful dieting tips to get rid of sugar. As a professional dietician and health consultant, I can only recommend you to take advantage of this free opportunity. People pay good money to hear this info from me in person. Anyhow, let's get into the sugary knowledge!

Examining Sugar

Sugar is a brief chain carbohydrate that is sweet and utilized as a part of the food. Most people know sugar as a whitish crystal-like powder with a sweet taste that is frequently added to everyday foods and beverages.

Sugar is also a common and plentiful product; a typical year sees millions of kilograms of table sugar delivered worldwide. The sugar that an average person consumes is experimentally termed as "sucrose," which separates into both glucose and fructose in the body. While sugar is an indispensable ingredient in numerous foods, many people have come to view it as harmful.

Research suggests that the human body does not need more than a single teaspoon of sugar at a given moment, and when it gets more than that (from sugar or starches that transform into sugar), here's what happens:

- Our blood sugar level rises (providing a brief "high").

- Our pancreas discharges insulin in light of the sugars/carbs we have consumed.

- Subsequently, the discharged insulin starts to take glucose from our circulatory system and convey it to our cells. We then crash and start to have a shaky feeling, tired or dizzy. It is the place where we go after more to recapture that sugar high, yet what they truly require is steadiness in their circulatory system.

- As our glucose level returns to the natural single teaspoon, the majority of the remaining glucose contributes to fat growth.

Even if you don't have a sweet tooth, many starchy foods can compound upon these health problems. Bagels, potato chips, and French fries are just a few examples. They're foods that contain "refined carbs," so they're equally problematic when it comes to continuing a cycle of unhealthy eating.

Sugar: Why Should You Avoid It?

- Sugar is an unfilled calorie - meaning it doesn't provide your body with any nutritional value whatsoever!
- Added sugar is not a required component of food, nor is it even suggested by nutritionists or doctors! There's a reason you don't see it on the food pyramid. Good starches, on the other hand, are definitely recommended, but sugar is not one of these.
- When we consume sugar, our body wastes energy handling the consumed molecules.
- Sugar lowers our immune system, making it difficult to battle off ailments. When we eat sugar-laden substances or beverages, we significantly disturb natural metabolic procedures. This makes it easier for the human body to get sick, and sometimes with serious conditions!
- Sugar stimulates the reward focus in your cerebrum – called the nucleus accumbens – to discharge dopamine, which causes an emotional high. That "awesome" feeling you

might get after eating a sugary product might not be all that healthy!

When you consume very sugary foods, an enormous amount of dopamine is discharged from the nucleus accumbens and this can cause addictive effects in high dosages. It's not far off from the possessive quality found in many prescription drugs.

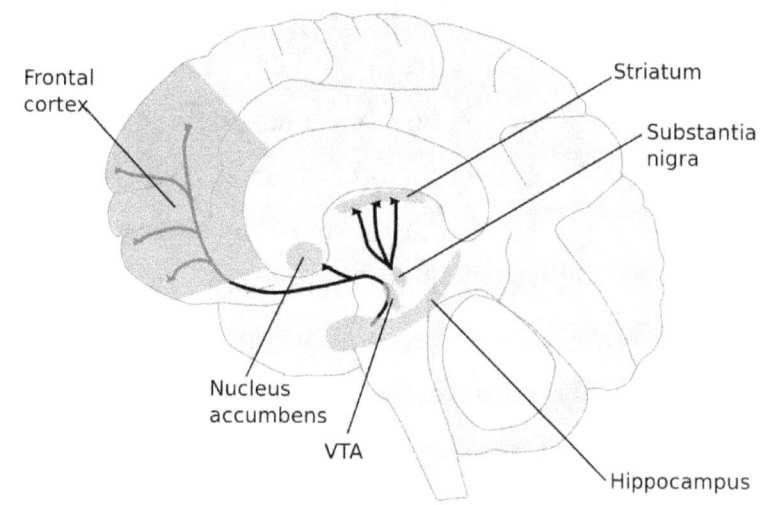

Dopamine Pathways in the Brain

The more sugar you consume, the more you eventually desire, as sugar causes a positive emotional impact through dopamine receptors. Sugar even works in a similar manner to cocaine or nicotine, which also provide emotional highs. For a few individuals, sugar even changes the brain's anatomy and its response to sugary foods, which eventually leads to a very ingrained addiction.

Addiction to flour and sugar is genuine, and it is not exclusively behavioural. It is a reported physiological issue that affects both your hormonal framework and your neurotransmitters. At Harvard, there have been recent academic studies, in which scientists found that extremely sugary milkshakes not only lead to a gigantic spike in glucose and insulin levels; they likewise stimulated enormous changes in brain activity.

To put it plainly, the brain ends up noticeably dependent on the energy spike from those milkshakes. This effectively makes added sugar no different from several illegal drugs, even if it doesn't seem as harmful.

The Difficulties in Dropping Sugar

Sugar addiction is no joke. Once addiction sets in, yearnings can be difficult to oppose, driving you down a dangerous slant towards obesity and other medical issues. Scientific studies are demonstrating that the human cerebrum can respond to sugar as it does to liquor or drugs.

This explains why you might feel down after initially cutting excessive sugars from your diet. When your body is burdened with waste, you feel awkward when not eating that specific food. Your body has also been physiologically conditioned towards sugary foods, so it might take some time to adjust to your new diet, both mentally and biologically.

However, your endeavor to reduce sugar will ultimately pay off. Individuals that undertake a sugar detox diet often see an improvement in their general vitality immediately and, after a brief timeframe, they also see a decrease in exhaustion. Additionally, the long-term advantages of curtailing excessive sugar in your eating routine are difficult to overlook.

An essay that was published in the diary *Circulation* demonstrated that sugar-sweetened beverages can lead to cardiovascular illness and diabetes, which results in roughly 184,000 individuals worldwide every year. Establishing a sugar detox routine means that you'll be all the more likely to avoid adding to that statistic.

Who Should Detox?

If you find yourself dependant on sugary foods for nourishment, or if your relationship to sugary foodstuffs is meddling with your lifestyle, then you may benefit from a sugar detox.

If you have diabetes — the continuum of metabolic harm ranging pre-diabetes to type two diabetes—or if you happen to have the Feel Like Crap (FLC) Syndrome, then detoxification can significantly enhance your wellbeing.

Sugar is the New Fat

Despite years of cultural indoctrination into believing that fat is terrible, many now believe that sugar, not fat, may also make you unwell and overweight.

The science is undoubted. Sugar, in all of its forms, is the main force behind our obesity pandemic. Sugar has also had a leading role in causing coronary illness, tumors, dementia, type two diabetes, depression, skin break outs, barrenness, ineptitude and a slew of other debilitating conditions.

It's not only destructive on a personal level; unhealthy eating has expanded into a full-blown, worldwide sociological issue. Only by pursuing healthy living, such as a sugar detox diet, can we ward ourselves from myriad health conditions.

Ten-Step Sugar Detox Plan

Apply the following 10 steps successfully and you will notice a significant change in you well-being, overall energy levels and hormone balance. I highly recommend to study the steps in detail and combine them with the chapters later on in this book.

Step 1: Remove All Sugar from Your Home

The least demanding approach to starting sugar detox without spending hours perusing labels is to dispose of anything that is bundled, canned, solidified (with the exception of a few special cases, as frozen natural berries) or pre-cooked. Even potato chips have sugar in them. There is such a large number of names for such a wide variety of sugar that it could take you a lifetime to weed them out by reading label after label, so sticking solely to whole foods is a guaranteed way of securing a healthy diet. Whole foods include products like nuts, eggs, poultry, seeds, meats, natural products, fish, and vegetables.

Step 2: Drink Unsweetened Beverages

Sugar in fluids is more hazardous for you than the sugar afforded by foods, as it enters your circulatory system very rapidly. The refreshment provided by sugary beverages doesn't last very long, so you're often tempted to drink successive beverages in a short period of time. Realize that drinks with heavy quantities of sugar aren't limited to soda or pop.

For example, a bottle of Gatorade contains fourteen teaspoons of sugar, which is about as much as a 20-ounce bottle of Coke. With all this sugar flying immediately into your circulatory system, the liver's fat-storage methods are hindered, prompting your body to produce extra fat within your stomach.

All sugar is half glucose (which increases sugar level in the blood) and half fructose. The latter is equivalent to the former when it comes to unhealthy eating, but often disregarded, wrongly, as less dangerous. Unless it can be metabolized and used as glucose, fructose can wreak havoc on the body. Ingesting considerable amounts of fructose causes your liver to release triglycerides into your circulatory system. A significant number of those triglycerides are likewise caught in your liver, which can with time prompt issues like "fatty liver ailments".

Step 3: Eat a High-Protein Breakfast

You've been fasting throughout the night, and that means that your carb levels are below average and your levels of insulin are high. This prompts many individuals to immediately reach for something sugary and tasty first thing in the morning. Counter this by eating a protein-heavy meal.

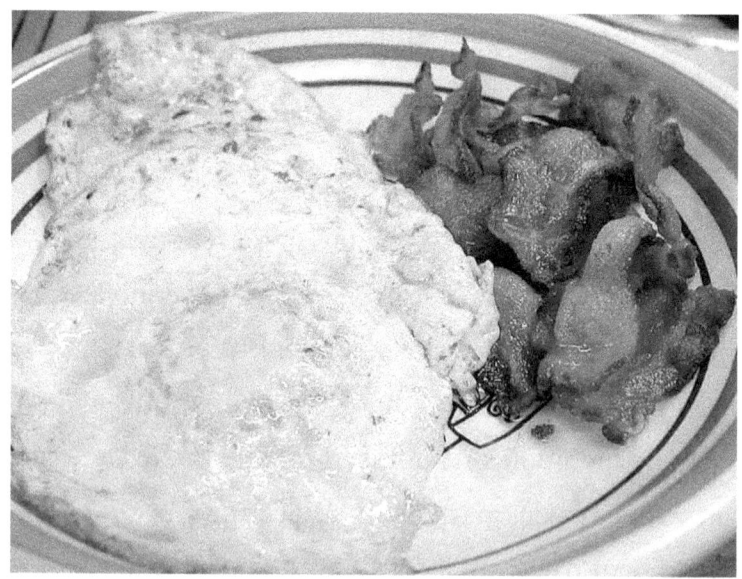

This will leave you feeling satisfied without causing your glucose to spike. It also encourages your body to use protein, not sugar, as your main source of energy from food. Be sure ingest sources of healthy fats on top of proteins. When you feel a craving for sugar, grab a protein shake, a few eggs, or a helping of walnuts instead.

Step 4: Look for Healthy Carbs

It should be noted that not every carb is the nutritional devil. Carbs are necessary for survival and optimal health. That being said, you should focus on consuming the healthiest sources of carbs possible, such as low-sugar veggies. Avoid white potatoes, corn, beets, winter squash, and sweet potatoes for the duration of the detox.

When you need something sweet, help yourself to fresh berries and fruits with low levels of sugar (plums, apples, and pears for example). Initially, during the beginning of your detox duration, you should not constrain your appetite by any means. Eat until your eyes fly out on the off chance that you need to. The entire crunch will fulfill you amid the initial few days of yearnings, and you might most likely drop a couple of pounds too.

Step 5: Eat Solid Fats

Fat is not to fault for physical heftiness – flour and sugar are. Fat steadies your glucose levels, keeps you feeling full, and transports vitamins and minerals throughout your system. You ought to have both fat and protein for each food you are eating.

The best sources of fats include nuts and seeds, nut margarine (except peanut butter), palm oil, coconut oil, olive oil, and avocados. Try to also include Omega-3 fats from meat, which you can get from pasture-raised meat, eggs, and wild fish.

Step 6: Keep Healthy Snacks Wherever You Can

It is as certain as Murphy's Law: you will get your most exceedingly awful yearnings when there is no an agriculturist's market, fruits stand, or healthy eatery within a five mile radius. Instead, there will most likely be five fast food eateries, three candy machines, and a doughnut shop in their place.

Be ready. Keep a lot of healthy snacks in your work area, in your automobile, in your laptop bag, and in any other place you can stash them. Rely on nuts, seeds, apples, jerky, celery with nut spread, berries and other convenient treats. It's best to have a blend of protein, carbs, and fats in each nibble.

Step 7: Lower Your Anxiety Level

Stress often makes many individuals search for comfort in sugary foods as a result of rising cortisol levels, which also bring about an increase in appetite and fat storage. It likewise meddles with your levels of leptin and ghrelin, the hormones that control craving and satiety. Take care to de-stress, which will naturally avert this process.

Various studies have demonstrated that simply doing some profound breathing can empower the Vagus nerve and change the concentration of your digestion from stowing away fat to processing it. Attend a class in fun fitness, take dancing lessons, call a friend for some conversation, watch an amusing video, have a pleasant bath, etc. Whatever it takes to de-stress – even if it's only for a couple minutes – will loosen you up and enhance your concentration.

Step 8: Lots of Sleep

A lack of sleep also raises your cortisol. Get no less than seven to nine hours of sleep every night. Many individuals find that doing this promotes fat reduction, enabling them to lose more weight without limiting their calorie intake.

Make sure you sleep for at least eight hours a night, in order to fulfil your resting habits. Recovery of the body is essential to get through the detox plan successfully, otherwise your body might hesitate to cooperate.

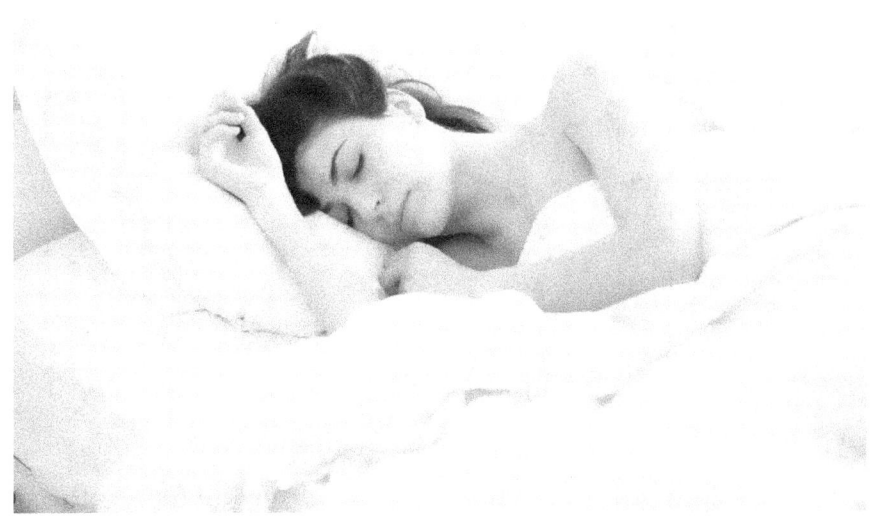

Step 9: Begin a Workout Plan

Strength workouts can assist you on your sugar detox and aid in keeping your glucose levels stable. When you utilize your muscles, they need more glucose, which drains your circulatory system of glucose and leads to fewer yearnings for sugary food.

This is especially true for thicker body types, but workouts are beneficial for everybody. Workouts also act as an excellent promoter of feel-good endorphins, leaving you less defenseless against mood eating.

Step 10: Minimize Inflammation

Inflammation brings about unhealthy glucose levels and prompts insulin resistance and Type 2 diabetes. However, disease or injuries are not to fault for most inflammatory cases – nourishment sensitivities are.

These are caused by issue foods like gluten and dairy, so remove them from your eating routine (if only for the initial detox days). You might not realize you suffered from either of these until several days into the detox. If you were previously susceptible to flares of inflammation, sugar detox should reliably reduce instances of gas, nausea, migraines, and bloating.

A sugar detox may appear somewhat outrageous to a few and sensible, though staggeringly hard to others. I guarantee you that this ten stage plan can help you effortlessly avoid sugar. The initial few days are the hardest, yet, with some persistence, you will feel great after a short period of time.

Let me give you some more motivation to start – the symptoms of sugar intake can have serious detrimental health effects, as we will explore in the next chapter. However, with the recipes in the last part of this book, you will be able to curb your sugar cravings into a more healthy habit.

Sugar Detox Symptoms

Notwithstanding the way that a few individuals claim to experience sugar withdrawals, the seriousness of any symptoms reported is questionable. The individuals who do not use sugar contend that regular sugar utilization can prompt mental health issues (for example, foggy thinking, attention issues, or hyperactivity).

Moreover, the risks of continuing to consume excessive amounts of sugar (especially when it comes to weight gain) are far greater than the risks of detox. Therefore, it is highly advisable to start your detoxification process as soon as you can despite the few minor symptoms that might occur.

It also appears as if sugar influences everybody in a very individualistic way – there are some who are more delicate to the side effects of sugar, while others may not see a lot of mental change from a sugar heavy diet versus going sugar-free. Whatever the case, here are a few side effects that have been reported by those undergoing sugar detox.

Variables That Impact Sugar Withdrawal

The following are a few variables that may impact your sugar detox: the length of your reliance on sugar, your normal day to day usage, your personal physiology, and whether you simply quit without any weaning period or slowly cut your consumption.

Time Span

How long have you been eating sugar on a regular basis? If you are similar to the vast majority sugar detox participants, you've likely been devouring sugar for the greater part of your life. Most normal eating regimes are loaded with sugar. The greater your consumption of sugary foods and drinks, the more difficult it will be to cut it from your diet entirely. Take care when beginning a sugar detox, it may be very difficult at the start!

Everyday Consumption

How much sugar do you eat each day? A few hundred years ago, the average American ate just around 2 pounds of sugar yearly. In the 1970's, that amount increased to 120 pounds annually. Nowadays, your normal American national ingests about 152 lbs. of sugar every year, or 3 pounds every week.

It is a truly exceptional change when contrasted with what individuals were eating in the 1800's. That being said, the less sugar you regularly devour, the simpler the withdrawal procedure will be. It will also reduce your chances of acquiring any severe side effects.

Personal Physiology

Everybody has a different reaction to sugar. Some individuals are very sensitive to its side effects, while others never suffer from any withdrawal symptoms. Thus, the difficulty in resisting cravings and other mental symptoms varies from person to person. This means that certain individuals can adjust to the impacts of cutting sugar from their eating regimes with greater speed than others.

While this may sound vague, and perhaps even disappointing to a few, understand that detoxification is a reality that's possible for everyone. Everybody can benefit from following the program, even if it takes some time to witness some initial results. After all – no pain, no gain!

Cold Turkey Versus Tapering

When beginning a diet plan, many quit sugar by simply stopping immediately, or going "cold turkey." This is no less effective than gradually weaning yourself off sugar, but realize that it can cause more pronounced withdrawal symptoms. Making such a significant biological and mental change to one's daily routine is undoubtedly going to cause some more articulated issues. It might be best to slowly cut your sugar intake over a period of 14 days.

By gradually decreasing the amount of sugar in your diet, you are slowly adjusting to this change, and it is thought to be a less demanding procedure. Both methods are equally effective, but going cold turkey can make the detox process much more jarring. Keep this in mind when you plan your diet.

Sugar Withdrawal Side Effects

The following are some conceivable side effects that you may encounter when you cut sugar from your eating routine. A longing for sugar and other starches is perhaps the most common manifestation of withdrawal.

Realize that not everybody will experience the majority of the side effects recorded beneath – withdrawal fluctuates in seriousness and intensity depending on the individual.

Outrage

If you stop cold turkey, your mood may plunge, and you may see that you are more irritable and angry than usual. The mood swings ought not to last more than two or three weeks, but it may make for a temporary shock.

Nervousness

Various people have reported uneasiness. Sugar can have an impact on dopamine levels and activity, which results in a susceptibility to jittery behaviour. Certain people will be sensitive than others when it comes to anxiety.

Changes in Appetite

Consuming sugar can lead to an amplified craving for carbohydrates. Moreover, when you quit devouring sugar, you may notice some changes in your overall appetite. However, it ought to return to normal after some time.

Cravings

A pining for sugar is the most evident impact of sugar withdrawal. They might even feel extraordinary and hard to overcome. So long as you remain disciplined, you will, in the long run, reach a point where these yearnings die down. It might help to remove all sources of sugar from your home, in addition to keeping sugar out of sight at all times. This will reduce the chances of you succumbing to those cravings.

Depression

Individuals may encounter a crash in mood. This mental plunge is typically not extreme, but may feel like symptoms of depression. Over the course of your detox, your mental state will rebalance.

Dizziness

In more outrageous instances of withdrawal, people have detailed feeling lightheaded upon discontinuing sugar. Though most individuals won't feel "dizzy" when they stop incorporating sugar in their eating regimes, some sensitive individuals may suffer from this unlikely effect.

Exhaustion

Sugar often provides a short term energy boost, so it is very typical to experience some broad weariness and torpidity amid the initial weeks of withdrawal. Over the long haul, an individual ought to return to normal levels of vitality.

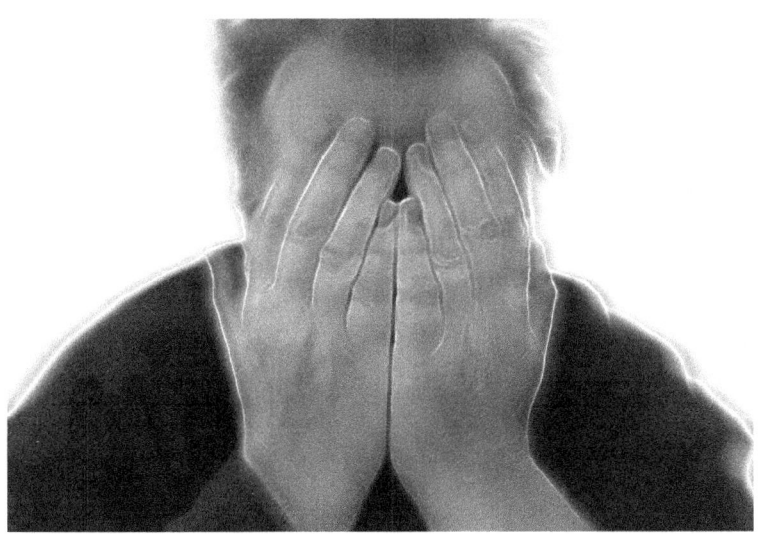

Flu-like Symptoms

At times, individuals encounter an extreme response sugar detox that results in low-grade flu-like symptoms. This outcome usually dies down within a couple of days. As with most of the other extreme scenarios, the vast majority of individuals will never experience this.

Migraines

Some participants have reported cerebral pains after beginning their diet. However, stress can also cause similar effects, and the biological changes caused by the diet may produce short-term migraines.

Trouble Sleeping

Dropping sugar from your eating routine may bring about brief upsets in patterns of sleep and arousal. You may notice that you cannot sleep at an appropriate time on account of restlessness. In a similar manner to the previously mentioned symptoms, this should disappear. Consider taking melatonin or engaging in a relaxing activity before bed if it becomes a major issue.

Irritability and Mood Swings

During the most intense period of your eating regimen, you may end up becoming snappy and irritable. Sugar can impact dopamine, which is one of the neurotransmitters in charge of pleasure in the mind. Other minor emotional episodes are a common occurrence.

These include minor depression, uneasiness, and other generally negative sentiments. Like the irritability, your emotional disposition will settle with patience, as your cerebrum takes some time to adjust to such a drastic change in diet. When someone suddenly removes the link between sugar and dopamine, some change in mood is to be expected.

Shaking

At times, individuals shake after radical diet adjustments. This is a genuinely normal and temporary symptom among individuals who quit eating sugar, and should subside shortly.

Weight Changes

Most individuals notice an improvement in fitness when they stop consuming sugar. Weight loss is one of the many reasons people engage in sugar detox.

Sugar Detox Duration: How Long?

There is no particular measure of time for the duration of sugar detox. The length of detox side effects and an improvement in health typically rely upon the individual undergoing the detox.

Some may see rapid physical and mental changes, while others may have a hard time combating sugar cravings. It completely depends on your current state of being, but also your health, age, and many other relevant factors. You would need a personal consult to determine your risks.

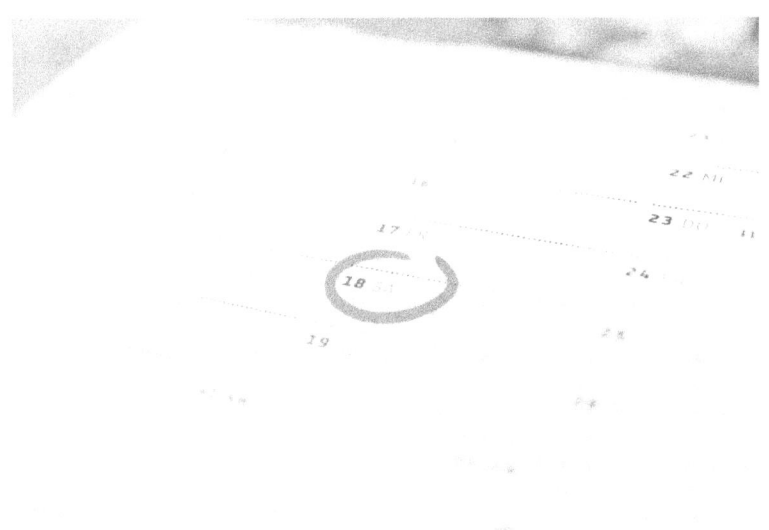

That being said, almost everyone suffers from some withdrawal symptoms, the length of which can vary. For some, the withdrawal symptoms were almost negligible and they felt remarkably better after only a few days. For others, it took nearly a month before they returned to a normal condition.

Withdrawal symptoms usually result from an imbalance in dopamine, which is often accompanied by a lack of sugar. In assisting in the addressing of this issue, it is prescribed to devour lean protein, fruits (blueberries and apples, for example), and nuts as nutritional supplements.

Whilst it might have to take some adaptations, getting through the first few days will help you find your new pattern of carb intake and will give your body some time to adapt. Expect some violent bowel movements and cravings along the way. It can be hard, but keep pushing to get into that healthy habit!

Getting Through Sugar Detox

Here's everything you have to think about while fighting detoxification symptoms. Removing unnecessary sugar from your diet is a great way of leading a healthy lifestyle, so keep these mental techniques in mind as you undergo detox.

Objective Setting is Your Friend

You may have heard of objective setting for personal goals and weight loss. However, shouldn't this technique be applied to sugar detox as well? It can be a standout among the best techniques for getting you through sugar detox. Treat yourself as a child if you must. When a child is told not to do something, they only desire to do it even more. They will do anything they can to go against an adult's wishes. Human minds simply do not care for the word no.

To overcome these instincts, you have to offer yourself motivation. Setting an objective or two will assist with that. When you give in to sugar cravings, you are preventing yourself from effectively achieving that objective.

Every moment you battle with a yearning is an opportunity to return to your objectives. What is so essential about them and why would you like to achieve them? Reminding yourself of a goal is a great way of preventing yourself from succumbing to an urge for sugar. Therefore sensible, practical goals are often vital for success in healthy living.

Your doctor may have warned you of a risk for diabetes. They may have warned you about an increase in weight, and the health dangers such a condition can pose. Perhaps you're simply tired of the rush/crash cycle that occurs when you devour sugar. Consider objectives and reasons that work in your favor. There is no point asking your companions what your objectives ought to be. If you believe in their judgment, be sure to get their advice before proceeding, but make the objectives and reasons individual and personal.

Keep Your Hunger at Bay

One of the ideal approaches battling sugar yearnings and withdrawal manifestations is to deny your body motivation to desire sugar. Bringing your appetite under control is an easy way to ensure this.

Realize that hunger is a common symptom. You will desire something terrible for you for its short term effects (it is cheap, common, and results in a boost of energy). All things considered, it won't give you enough vitality for the duration of the day.

Concentrating on a balanced, healthy diet will ensure that you do not fall upon sugar as a way to boost energy. This can be done in several ways. Here's what I always recommend.

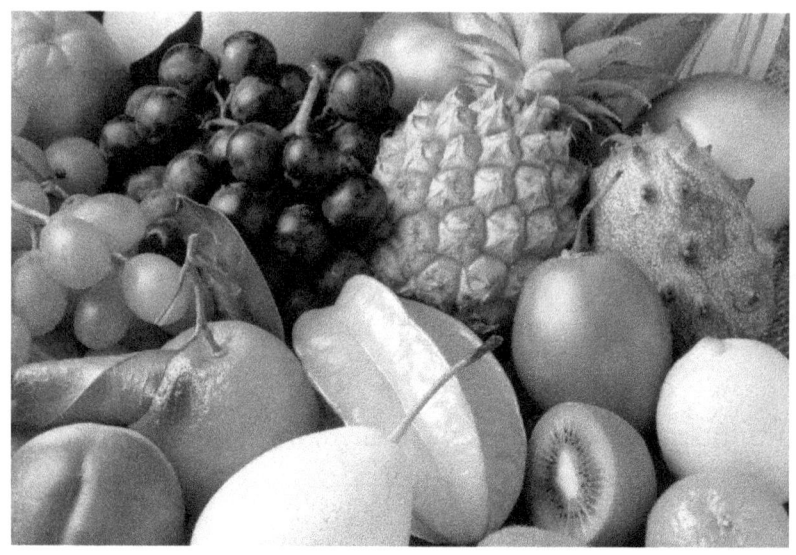

Ensure you have your three huge meals or six little meals—whichever manner you like to eat—over the course of the day. If you choose to eat three large meals, keep a few snacks on hand.

When your appetite is under control, you should feel changes in your perception of eating. After all, there is no requirement for your cerebrum to begin instructing you to eat overly sweet things. In any case, what will you replace those sweets with? You have to eat something besides sugary foods, correct?

Find Naturally Sweet Foods

Switch bars of chocolate for fruit and yogurt. They might not seem as tasty, but you'll acquire natural sugar from them as opposed to overloaded, unnatural sugar. Your mind still processes these foods as sugary products. Unlike artificially added sugar, the sugar from natural products is discharged into your body over time. You will not feed an immediate high, and you will not receive a sudden release of insulin.

This means you also won't feel a crash when that sugar leaves your system. Organic products, like fruits, are also brimming with fiber and vitamins, keeping you feeling full for a longer duration. One nibble will last you until your next meal, and will also keep you from aggressively snacking. Furthermore, this trick works for more than just snacks. You can add naturally sweet food into full meals.

Try including ginger or lemon juice in larger dishes. Cinnamon, coriander, and nutmeg are also excellent choices. As they all have sweet tastes, they replace the foods your body typically takes as sugars.

With regards to dessert, help yourself to a fruit salad with pineapples, mangos, and melons. Natural yogurt is another healthy option, especially when combined with lemon squeeze and nutmeg. These options not only trick the mind; they feel satisfyingly sweet enough to function as a treat after a long day.

Balance Glucose in Your Diet

Even naturally sweet foods result in some glucose. Including more fats, fibers, and proteins is a great way of managing your glucose levels.

Keep in mind that the body breaks down protein and fiber gradually. You won't excessive consume calories from foods rich with fibers and protein because they do not cause a reaction as glucose does. Yet, how does the fat offer assistance?

First, the body requires fat for a healthy mind, particularly omega three and other unsaturated fats. Fats also assist with the absorption of vitamins. Consuming fats will help you attain a healthy body, one that supports all vital organs. They also help the body feel full, further preventing cravings. Attempt to eat more dairy products, such as cheddar, to give your body the fats it needs.

Rehydrate

Dehydration can be a big issue. Not exclusively does it keep your organs from functioning properly, but it also influences your cerebrum and the yearnings it could potentially cause.

You will endure more cerebral pains, causing more withdrawal side effects. Dehydration can also lead to hunger. So it's essential to keep your body full of that wet, watery substance.

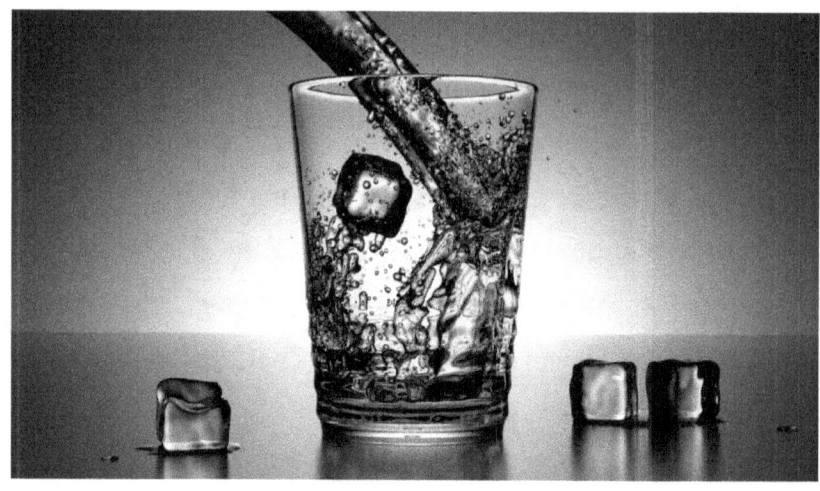

Your mind cannot differentiate between a craving for food and thirst. When you are dehydrated, your stomach will instead transmit the message that you are hungry. It may push you to devour a huge amount of calories, well above your daily requirements.

Try drinking a glass of water whenever you feel a yearning for something sweet. You can even include a few cuts of lemon or cleaved strawberries to give your water a naturally sweet taste. Be sure to avoid artificial sweeteners or fruit juices. Water takes up space in the stomach, so it may prevent you from feeling hungry until a proper mealtime. Try not to drink excessively. Furthermore, do not supplant meals with water. You will risk numerous medical issues in doing so. If you still feel hungry a few minutes after drinking a glass of water, you probably need a full meal! Go after a healthy dinner or lunch, and not something sweet to tide you over.

Distract Your Brain

Cravings for sugar will often come when you are not active. For those attempting to get thinner, boredom eating may be a serious issue. It worsens your sugar withdrawal symptoms and keeps you going after those tasty snacks.

However, it is a great opportunity to find a way how to keep your brain from sugar yearnings. The more you ignore them, the less impact they will have on you. Engage in an activity or hobby that you've been itching to do.

As you discover satisfaction in something else, your cheerful hormones will rise, and you will not feel as restless or depressed over the absence of sugar.

When you're staring at the TV or doing something else that can prompt nibbling, keep your hands occupied. A few ladies have found sewing or croqueting helps. They can glue their eyes on the screen still enjoy their favorite programs, while they busy their hands. Their brains are removed from frequent calls for those seductive sugary treats.

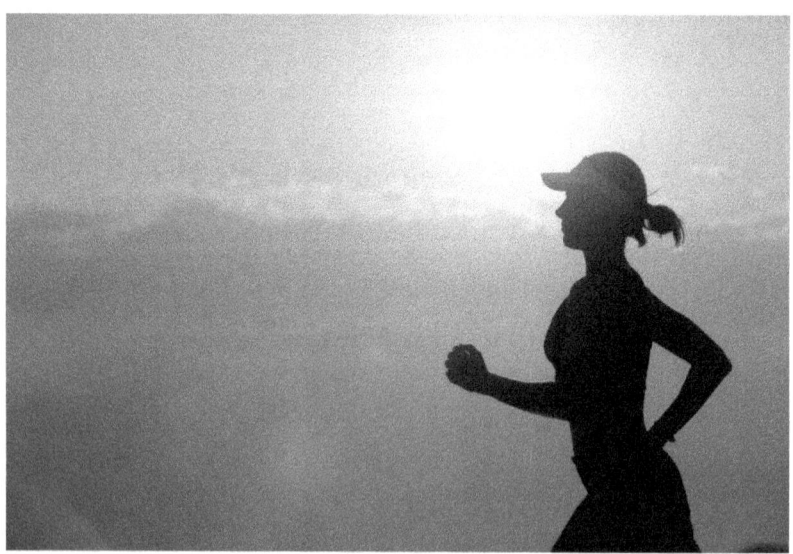

Working out is a fabulous approach to conquering longings and detox symptoms. Getting some exercise enhances the body's serotonin and endorphins. This makes it an incredible approach to battling gloom and nervousness, and will likewise dispose of muscular painfulness and migraines.

In finding a workout that you truly cherish doing, you will discover that your mind benefits in a lot of ways. You are not forcing yourself to accomplish something. All the more great hormones will be discharged, and you will feel encouraged to continue. Additionally, your mind is removed from worry during exercise. You discover the detox symptoms simpler to deal with since you cannot remember they exist!

Fuel Yourself With Sleep

You have fuelled your body with the correct food and you are ensuring that you protect the body with workouts. The next step is uncovering approaches towards fuelling the mind. Protecting your cerebrum has several long-term effects. A well-fuelled cerebrum will combat yearnings, sadness, and all of those other irritating detox symptoms.

How can you accomplish that?

Sleeping more is a good start.

This is easier said than done. Recall that a sleeping disorder is one of the indications of sugar withdrawal. When you sleep, you may have some insane dreams preventing you from achieving a full night's rest. So, how can you go about conquering these symptoms?

You can begin by keeping yourself to a schedule. Go to bed at the same time every night and get up at the same time every day. This goes a long way in reducing withdrawal symptoms. Your insomnia and strange dreams will turn into relics of a time long past. It also aids in relaxing both the psyche and the body. Take a relaxing shower, sit down with a book, or listen to calming music that helps you nod off. With more rest comes a healthier cerebrum. You will resist melancholy and anxiety, in addition to all the other undesirable withdrawal symptoms.

Keep It Simple

Going on a sugar-free eating regimen is pointless if you are underprepared. The most appropriate thing you can do is: get everything out of your kitchen cupboards that contains sugar—and be sure to read the fine print!

Go through the packaging and expel anything that makes the detox process more difficult. Fill your pantries and cooler with nutritious goodness. Porridge oats may seem flat, yet you can include a few fruits for natural flavor.

The simpler you make the process for yourself, the less demanding the detox stages will seem.This is your opportunity to concentrate on a more beneficial way of life. Of course, that doesn't mean it's going to be easy. Withdrawal, motivation, and craving are all obstacles on your path to a better you. Make it simple yourself to adjust by curbing any temptations and actively disposing of unhealthy products.

By taking after the tips above, you won't stress over the risk of eating an excessive amount of sugar. You will remain focused on getting all the supplements your body requires and experience a long and glad life. But there's a ton of more advantages. Let's explore some of them.

The Advantages of Sugar Detox

By picking up the sugar detox program, you will start earning a large number of stunning advantages that you do not have the capacity to accomplish any other way. There are nine great reasons that you ought to begin this program of sugar detox for yourself.

Reduced Appetite

Sugar can make you eat more than you ought to. Sugar's influence over the cerebrum impacts its ability to gauge appetite levels. You end up overeating and devouring more high-fructose meals. The more sugar you consume on a normal day, the more you consume with every meal. This causes an increase in weight, not to mention a languid feeling.

As you move through the steps of sugar detox, your cravings will gradually diminish, leaving you more capable of adhering to a good diet. This is far from the only advantage, however.

Weight Loss

As you might expect, a reduction in appetite leads to a reduction in weight, which is what draws many to the sugar detox program in the first place. Obesity, which is common for those that eat large amounts of added sugar, can result in an enormous amount of medical problems. Sugar consumption encourages the body to store devote unused energy to fat cells, which leads to weight gain.

Sugar detox helps regulate the body and reduce an overabundance of fat that you may have accumulated. Over the course of the program, you will keep on seeing changes in your as you proceed with your newly discovered dietary patterns.

More Energy

Eating excessive amounts of sugar may have caused problems you were previously unaware of. Weight gain leads to laziness and sluggish energy levels, making it difficult to accomplish anything. This is one of the main motivations you ought to consider before beginning the sugar detox framework, as you will see this change in just a couple days.

As sugar starts to deplete from your body, you will feel a surge of vitality. You will find yourself able to dedicate more time to activity and exercise. While you keep on following the sugar detox framework and workout you won't just shed more weight than you thought conceivable; energy, too, can increase by leaps and bounds. This is pleasing both in the moment and long term, and enriches every day of your detox program.

Mood Improvement

While many individuals go after pails or tubs of dessert to help with handling their hardships, they negatively impact their bodies in doing so. Yes, consuming these sugar stashed treats can make you feel pleased for a brief moment, as this releases a burst of dopamine into the cerebrum. Nonetheless, after you quit consuming sugar, those levels of dopamine drop, thereby dragging the body into a spiral of despair that leads them to consume yet another tub of dessert. Avoiding an imbalance of mood is the fourth reason for choosing a sugar detox diet.

You may feel a little crumby in the beginning. Nevertheless, after some time, your state of mind will begin to brighten. Your body will start to conform to the absence of dopamine in your framework and permit you to appreciate bliss without the guide of sugar. If you happen to feel the despondency incurred by sugar consumption and withdrawal, your dejection will gradually fade away all through the detox procedure, turning you into a significantly more joyful and healthier you.

Healthier Skin

Your skin might be a great deal more dry and fragile than it ought to be, as sugar adds to droopy skin and wrinkles. You may not see the expansion or the distinction in your skin as fast as you would your weight or an absence of energy. However, it happens each time you eat a piece of candy. Sugar deactivates the antioxidants in your body, as well as enhances the impact that the sun has upon the skin.

All through the sugar detox procedure, your body will start to redress the harm that has been caused by your sugar binging. Soon, you may start to look more youthful, and your appearance will be extraordinarily enhanced over the days you have committed to the detox. The collagen in your skin will start to mend itself to give you substantially lovelier, healthier skin. Remember that this will require some time investment and persistence, but the result makes it an important reason for following sugar detox guidelines.

Better Digestive Health

Numerous sugary foods swell your digestive framework. While this swelling causes gas and queasiness in a few individuals, other people never even notice this occurring inside their bodies. The distress that you experience in the wake of eating a substantial meal or sugary snack can often be attributed to digestive swelling. It may even cause you to vomit, which is unhealthy on top of being awkward.

Sugar detox frees the digestive system from being chafed and swollen by sugar. Your intestines and stomach will process food smoothly, without causing a swollen feeling. You'll be able to enjoy meals more, and your digestive system will thank you for pursuing the healthier choice.

Better Circulation

Everybody knows how imperative their circulatory framework is. Sugar brings an overabundance of insulin within your circulation system, which prompts expanded growth of the veins. The walls and arteries of vessels stiffen as they grow quicker than expected. This may eventually put you at risk for heart issues. The strained quality of blood vessel walls (especially in the arteries) are prone to causing serious conditions, such as a stroke, if they are placed under pressure.

While this bodily response to sugar appears to be irreversible, a sugar detox can gradually correct this. The rate at which the walls of your blood vessels develop will return to ordinary levels, and walls will start to sufficiently thin and flex when pressure is applied. This can diminish your risk of strokes and heart issues. Nonetheless, you should watch out for your sugar utilization to evade dipping back into dangerous levels.

Diminished Health Risks

If you managed to get to a specialist before starting the sugar detox process, they will presumably disclose that you are at hazard for a large number of various medical issues. The eighth motivation behind sugar detox is precisely that: bringing down your risk for serious medical illness. There are numerous issues caused by consuming an abundance of sugar every day. You put yourself at a risk of diabetes, as well as circulatory and heart conditions. These are risks that are life threatening and ought to be dealt with a lot of seriousness and care.

Sugar detox can help remedy your unfortunate dietary patterns by bringing down your glucose levels and hauling you off the beaten path of numerous medical problems. These developments will not guarantee perfect health. However, the practices you will learn throughout the detox procedure will assisting you in remaining healthy and avoiding unhealthy habits as much as possible. While many individuals may not understand the issues sugar can bring to their wellbeing, others have contacted specialists, who have suggested diminishing in their sugar utilization.

Lower Cholesterol Levels

A high level of cholesterol is the last reason someone might undergo a sugar detox. High cholesterol is another trait behind diabetes. Numerous sugary foodstuffs have large amounts of cholesterol, and the liver can't sift through everything, leaving you with a high chance of getting cholesterol issues.

Sugar detox brings down both your glucose and your cholesterol levels. As you set up each of your meals, you will discover the delight in preparing foods and dishes free of cholesterol. Bringing down your cholesterol level and sugar admission will give you more vitality, health, and joy that you would have ever thought conceivable.

Break Free from Food Enslavement

Detoxing inverts the food dependence that is brought on by the trillion-dollar mechanical sustenance framework—the infrastructure that transforms sugar, salt, and fat into medication-like food that ensnares you with each chomp. This constant flow of hyper-prepared, exceedingly sugary, and seriously addictive nourishments attacks your cerebrum chemistry, your health, and your waistline. As though food enslavement is not sufficiently damaging by itself, the modern industrial foods that contain this drug-like impact can likewise prompt serious bodily concerns, like diabetes.

The best approach to recover your life and your well-being begins with what is typically known as rehab. It may prove for some intense changes, yet it will give you the ability to assist you in getting thinner, changing your organic chemistry, and in doing away with your addiction until the end of time. Our taste buds, waistlines, mind chemistry, and digestion have been hijacked by the food industry. The sugar detox diet assists us in recovering health and breaking free from the industry of food that has cash, not well-being, as its main concern.

Save Cash

Lamentably, we have been deluded into assuming that eating sound is costly as truly overrated processed nourishment kept us fat and depleted our financial balance. An unhealthy lifestyle leads to more sick days and more visits to the doctor, which further diminishes your income. The sugar detox diet assists your income in quick ways. If you are requesting an order of take out on Friday evenings, you might be shocked to find that cooking your particular food can spare you cash. By rearranging your financial plan and investigating other superfluous optional spending, you may make all the more cash for good sustenance.

Satisfying Sex

I wager you weren't expecting this one. However, sex hormones and insulin adjustments are more connected than you might expect. Many believe that a low sex drive is simply a consequence of aging.

It is not. Maturing doesn't require men and women to reach after pills to satisfy their sexual activity. Unhealthy habits (drinking and smoking, for instance) and a stressful environment can lead to very imbalanced sex hormones. When you undertake the sugar detox diet, you wipe out poisonous substances in the body (and, as we've demonstrated, sugar is equivalent to debilitating drugs) that ruin your hormonal balance.

When you realize how insulin can affect different hormones (counting your sex hormones), it's easy to draw an obvious conclusion as to how sugary food can limit your sexual life.

6 Healthy Sugar Detox Recipes

Here's some good ideas for your to get inspired eating better. It's by no means a comprehensive guide – more an inspirational few meals to get you going. Go ahead and try them, I eat some of these delicious meals quite a few times a month!

Breakfast #1: An English Muffin with Peanut Butter and Jelly

Alternative: Avocado on Sprouted Bread

We adore a decent peanut butter and jelly sandwich, yet finding locally acquired nutty spread without added sweetness (which frequently comes as Palm natural product oil) can get challenging.

Make certain to examine ingredients keenly and search for a nut margarine that is made with nothing but with nuts, a little sea salt, and oil. Or consider having avocado on toast. The high-fat substance in avocado keeps you feeling full, while sprouted grants vitamins, minerals, and fiber. Stylize your avocado toast with lime squeeze, a dash of red pepper pieces, or cayenne pepper. You can likewise top it with a poached egg for more protein.

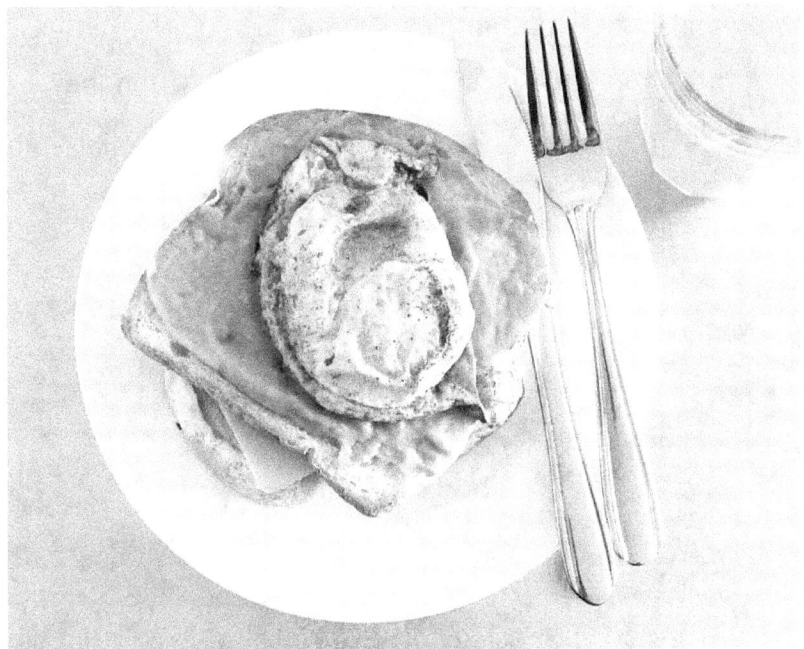

Breakfast #2: Almond Milk and Whole-Grain Cereal

Alternative: Overnight Oats with Berries

Unless you happen have a dairy-free diet or are trying to reduce your intake of soaked fat, realize that a lot of soy milk, rice milk, and nut milk contain heaps of added sugar. Instead, go for unsweetened renditions. Keep in mind that most "solid" locally acquired cereals tout containing oats, quinoa, and other entire grains, though they are regularly spiked with honey, molasses, darker rice syrup, and different sweeteners.

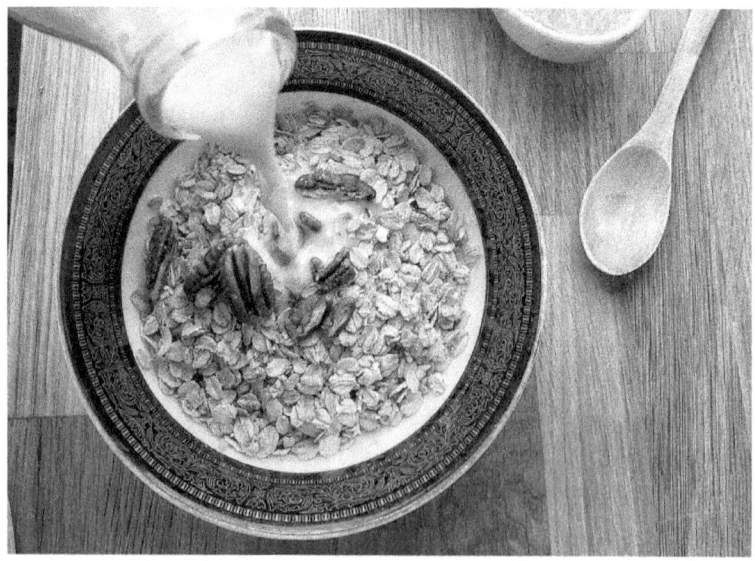

Instead, try a handcrafted breakfast and overnight oats. Just blend some unsweetened almond milk with a half a mug of steel-cut oats and a bit of 2% plain Greek yogurt. Do not forget to include chia seeds to make the blend thick, alongside nuts, new berries, vanilla concentrate, and ground cinnamon to inject some flavor.

Lunch #1: Grilled Cheese and Tomato Soup

Alternative: Lentil Soup and Lettuce-Wrapped Turkey Sandwich

I hate to be the one to break it to you, but ketchup, pasta sauces, and tomato-based soups have sugar stowing away in the ingredients. Your most solid alternative: make your own "sauce" by pureeing cooked tomatoes, including minced garlic and naturally ground pepper for taste.

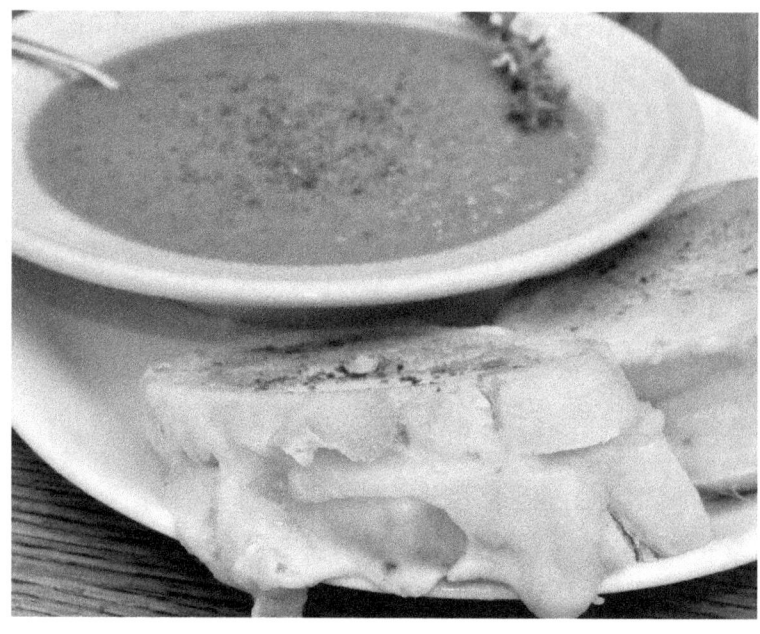

Even better, attempt a turkey lettuce wrap with flame-broiled cheddar and tomato soup. Throw in a cut of provolone, olives, or tomatoes. As an afterthought, settle for lentil soup — a great veggie lover wellspring of protein and fiber — to keep you satisfied and control longings.

Lunch #2: Broccoli Salad, Dried Cranberries

Alternative: Salmon Salad with Lemon-Olive Oil Dressing

Do not give the broccoli a chance to trick you! While a conventional broccoli serving of mixed greens seems healthy with bacon bits, cheddar pieces, red onions and cherry tomatoes, the dressing frequently requires a quarter measure of sugar. (Correct, sugar).

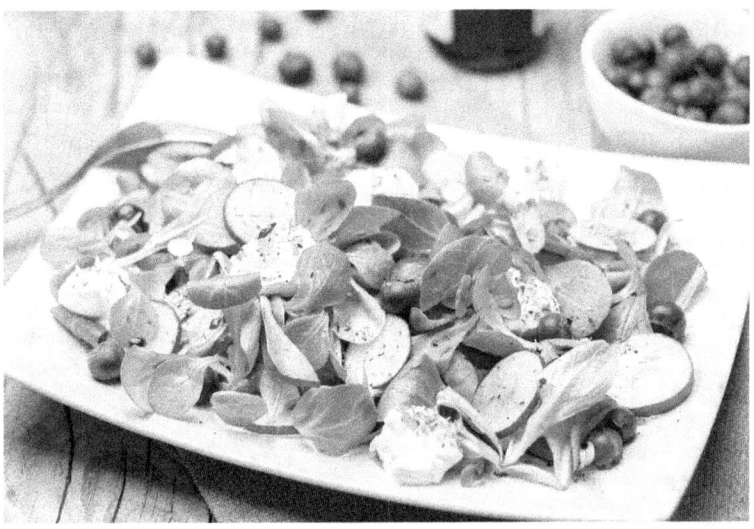

Those grams of sugar shoot up significantly when you include dried cranberries to the blend. For a better adjusted lunch, set up a serving of salmon with mixed greens (a great source of omega-3 unsaturated fats and lean protein) with crisp berries for a touch of sweetness. Hurl it in a basic lemon juice, ocean salt, and EVOO dressing, and you're ready to go!

Supper #1: Barbecue Chicken, Baked Beans

Alternative: Rotisserie Chicken that has a Cannellini Bean Salad

This may appear like a harmless dinner, yet many grill sauces, along with maple syrup and ketchup, have walloping measures of sugar. Fiber can also be found in baked beans.

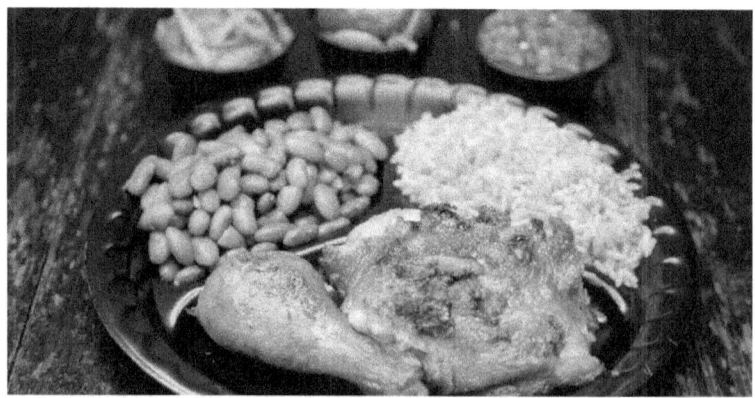

As another option, get a rotisserie chicken ready for a speedy supper and present it with a crisp cannellini bean salad of mixed greens made with cut new basil, lemon juice, EVOO and salt, and pepper to taste.

Supper #2: Mashed Potatoes, Teriyaki Tuna

Alternative: Sweet Potatoes and Pepper-Crusted Tuna Steak

Teriyaki sauce sounds innocuous. However, it is made with mirin — a Japanese wine that is sweet — white sugar, honey, or corn starch. Put those together and you may as well have a doughnut for supper.

It actually looks delicious, and there's so few carbs in this meal! With the Japanese influences you will feel like you're dining in an Asian restaurant.

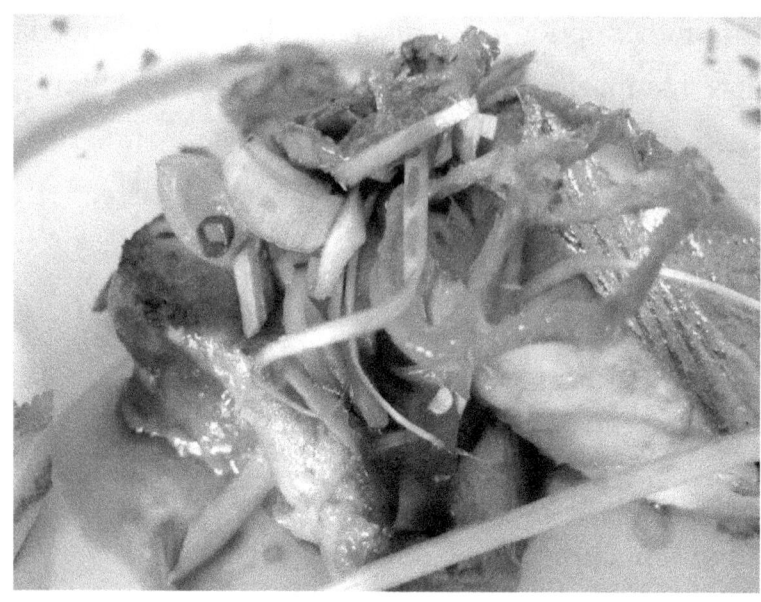

Substitute teriyaki sauce with a low-sodium soy sauce imbued with lemon juice, hacked crisp parsley, oregano and minced garlic. While white potatoes do have healthy advantages, sweet potatoes work just as well as a side dish to cut sugar cravings, since they're sweet and have a high degree of fiber.

Detoxing Your Body

The outcomes are unfathomable. This is not just a detox program, it's a healthy way of life. After one realizes and experiences the beneficial outcomes, they will proceed with a sugar-free lifestyle.

It is not a health improvement plan or a 3-day detox program. Rather, it's an instructive, straight forward and a practical set of guidelines to remove sugar out of your life, so you can appreciate every one of the advantages that accompany it.

I trust we, as a whole, ought to change our eating regimens and dispose of added sugar, as it is the bedrock of the greater part of our sustenance and medical issues. Added sugar is the real reason for some pestilence, and it ought to be your main concern.

So, yes, I am a fan of no added sugar that needs to transform the world, and who trusts that a low-sugar world is conceivable. However, we instruct individuals to pursue this goal. When we know about the issue we as a whole can roll out the improvements in ourselves.

Parting Words

With these final words, this short guidebook on the sugar detox diet comes to a conclusion. We have looked at the entire process, from root causes to solutions, and everything in between. I have thoroughly enjoyed creating this short guidebook, and I hope you have learned something from it!

If you feel like you want to know more, make sure to grab the **free bonus ebook** with 21 sugar dieting tips I wrote for the people that are committed to learn more. Get it immediately mailed to you, by going to my website on this specific page:

http://www.stephanygreene.site/free-ebook

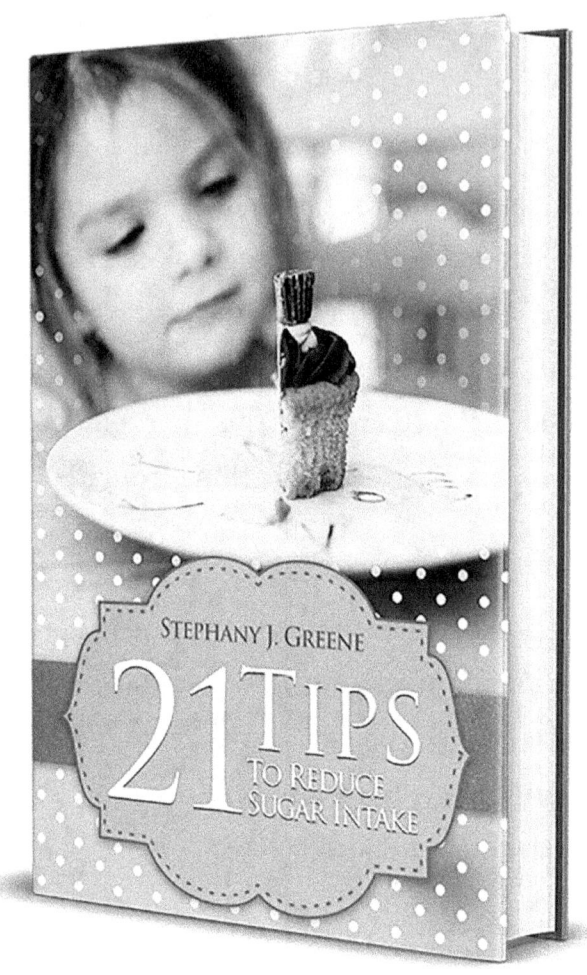

Changing your lifestyle in any way is often a difficult and time-consuming thing. However, the results can be very rewarding, even when it comes to the little things. By now, you know what foods to avoid and which ones to embrace: a long process of change awaits you with this newly found knowledge.

Start Today

Making a start is 50% of the work, I truly believe that. Once you make the shift in your mindset, actively wanting to change your life for the better, is a profound decision that will help you on your path to a healthier life.

I also highly recommend picking up my extensive guide on intermittent fasting, a book I wrote for people looking to live a healthier and more natural lifestyle, whilst not changing around their diet a lot. You can pick up the book by simply searching on Amazon for "Intermittent Fasting Stephany Greene". You will not be disappointed by picking up that guide, because it will completely change the way you think about dieting.

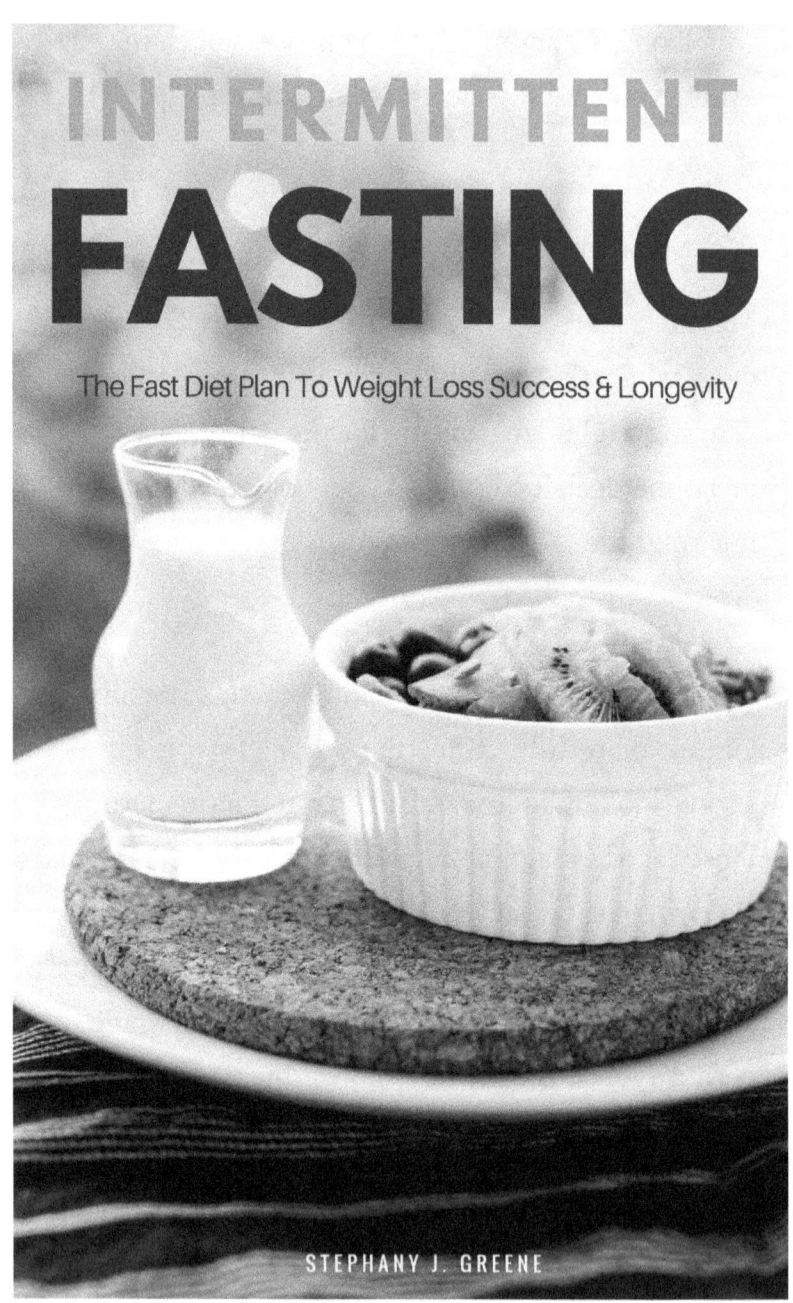

INTERMITTENT
FASTING

The Fast Diet Plan To Weight Loss Success & Longevity

STEPHANY J. GREENE

For now, I wish to sincerely thank you for your time spent reading this book. It was a great pleasure to create, and hopefully also a great pleasure to read. Best of luck to you and make sure to keep an eye out for some of the sugar diet-related books I'm about to publish in the near future. If you've downloaded my free ebook, you will likely be notified by e-mail about my upcoming books in the near future. So make sure to look out for some messages from me, and if you do not get them, make sure to check your spam folder as well. Thanks and best of luck!

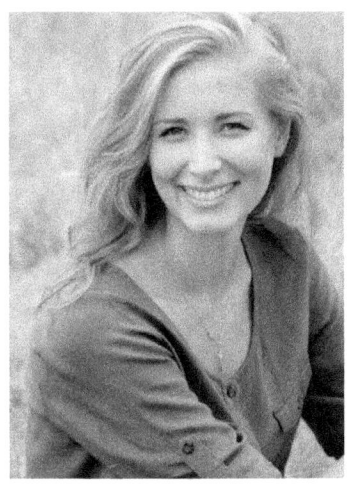

Stephany J. Greene

Author & Dietician

www.ingramcontent.com/pod-product-compliance
Lightning Source LLC
Chambersburg PA
CBHW071228280526
45787CB00002B/845